100 MINI WEIGHT LOSS TIPS

USEFUL ADVICE FOR THOSE WHO WANT TO LOSE WEIGHT
PERMANENTLY

BY:

I0435533

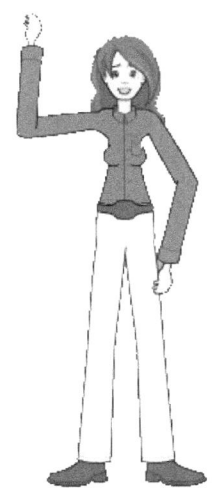

MARIA MARKELLA
(INDEPENDENT RESEARCHER, HEALER, ADVISOR & AUTHOR)
MARIAMARKELLA@YAHOO.COM

HAVE A LOOK AT MORE OF BOOKS FROM MARIA:
HTTP://AMAZON.COM/AUTHOR/MARIAMARKELLA/

ISBN-13: 978-1499274431

ISBN-10: 1499274432

DISCLAIMER: ALTHOUGH THE AUTHOR HAS PUT ALL HER EFFORTS TO PRESENT FRESH AND VALID INFORMATION TO THE READER, DUE TO THE CHANGING NATURE OF THE SUBJECT OF WEIGHT LOSS, THE AUTHOR CANNOT GUARANTEE ANY SUCCESS IN LOSING WEIGHT.

PRINTED BY CREATESPACE, AN AMAZON.COM COMPANY

INTRO

FOOD IS IMPORTANT. IN FACT, FOOD IS THE ONLY SUBJECT EVERYONE CAN TALK ABOUT. MAYBE IT IS THE MOST DISCUSSED SUBJECT WORLDWIDE. IN THIS BOOK I WILL SHARE MY BEST 100 WEIGHT LOSS TIPS.

GATHERING ALL THE ADVICE TOOK ME ALMOST 1 YEAR. I HOPE YOU ENJOY THE END RESULT. IF YOU DO ENJOY THIS BOOK, PLEASE LEAVE A POSITIVE REVIEW ON AMAZON.

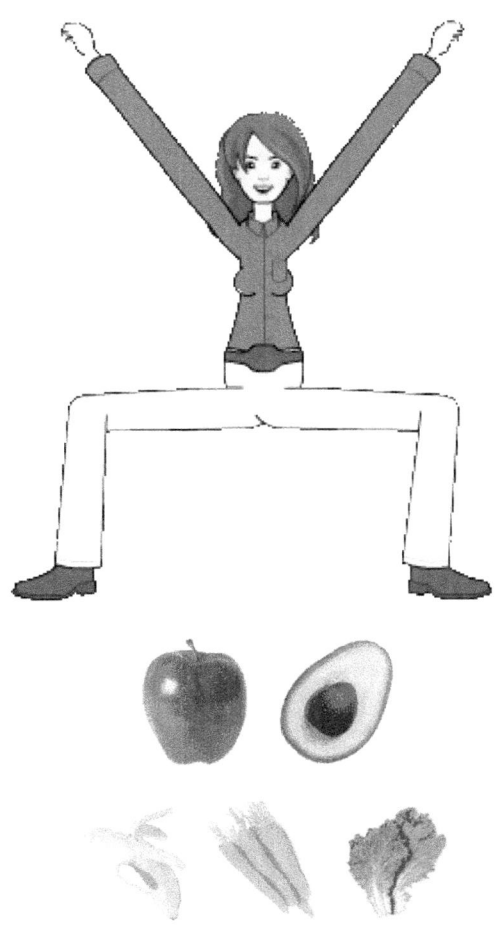

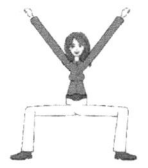

[WEIGHT LOSS TIPS 1 - 5]

1

CONSIDER THE DIFFERENT HEALTHY WAYS OF COOKING, APART FROM FRYING STUFF. THERE IS ROASTING, STEAMING, BAKING AND MORE.

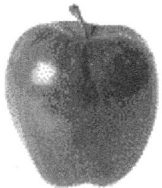

2

IN MOST RESTAURANTS THERE ARE CERTAIN FOODS THAT COME BEFORE THE MAIN MEAL AND AFTER THE MAIN MEAL. FOCUS ON THE MAIN MEAL AVOIDING ANYTHING ELSE THAT SEEMS UNHEALTHY.

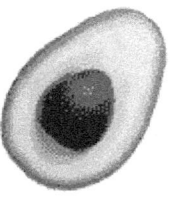

3

BRING AUTOMATION INTO YOUR EATING. PLAN YOUR MEALS BEFORE-HAND. THIS IS A GREAT WAY TO AVOID MAKING A BAD FOOD CHOICE DURING THE DAY.

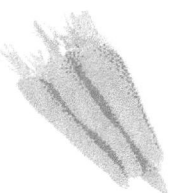

4

SINCE YOU PROGRAM YOUR MEALS IT IS RECOMMENDED THAT YOU AVOID SKIPPING A MEAL. IT WILL MAKE YOU FEEL "EMPTY" AND UNHAPPY.

5

STRESS LEADS TO MORE EATING. THIS IS WHAT SCIENCE TELLS US. TRY TO FIGHT STRESS WITH MEDITATION OR SIMILAR ALTERNATIVE TREATMENT.

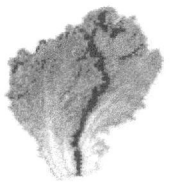

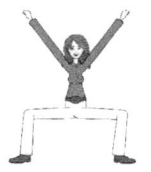

[WEIGHT LOSS TIPS
6 – 10]

6

OAT IS A GREAT FRIEND OF YOURS. IF YOU EAT A GOOD MEAL WITH OAT IN THE MORNING IT WILL KEEP YOU STRONG THE WHOLE DAY.

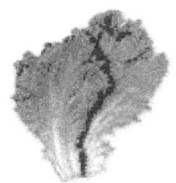

7

ADD OLIVE OIL, FISH (SALMON IS MY BEST) AND WALNUTS TO YOUR DIET. YOU WILL FEEL STRONG AND WITH A SENSE OF SATISFACTION.

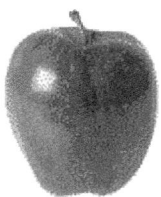

8

WHEN YOU GO GROCERY SHOPPING, HAVE A LIST (OF THE ITEMS YOU NEED) PREPARED BEFORE-HAND TO AVOID BEING DISTRACTED BY UNHEALTHY FOODS IN THE SHELVES.

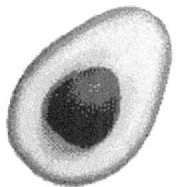

9

INCLUDE A GREEN SALAD TO YOUR MAIN MEALS. USE LEMON (OR VINEGAR) TO DRESS THE SALAD. IT WILL HELP YOU ABSORB THE NUTRITIOUS FOOD STUFF EASIER.

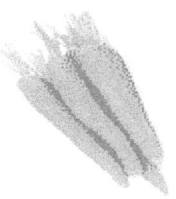

10

SOMETIMES PEOPLE CONFUSE HUNGER WITH THIRST. WHEN YOU FEEL YOU NEED TO EAT SOMETHING, TRY DRINKING SOME WATER FIRST.

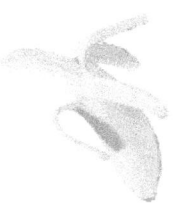

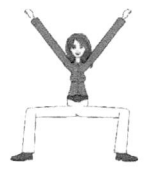

[WEIGHT LOSS TIPS
11 – 15]

11

EATING NUTS FREQUENTLY IS A GREAT CHOICE. NUTS WILL MAKE YOU
FEEL "FULL". YOU CAN EAT THEM AFTER YOU SOAK THEM IN WATER OR
MILK.

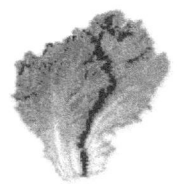

12

THIS MIGHT SOUND WEIRD BUT PUT YOUR FOOD IN SMALL PLATES.
YOU MAY DISCOVER THAT A CHILDREN'S PLATE IS MORE APPROPRIATE
FOR AN ADULT WHO WANTS TO LOSE WEIGHT...

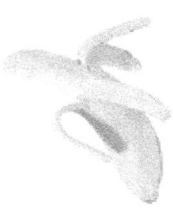

13

YOU CAN REPLACE FOOD WITH SEX. INVITE YOUR LOVER (IF YOU HAVE
ONE) AND ENJOY THIS BEAUTIFUL ACTIVITY. IT WILL ALSO BOOST YOUR
SELF-CONFIDENCE.

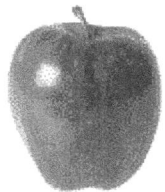

14

YOU SHOULD DO YOUR OWN "FOOD STYLING" WHEN PREPARING YOUR MEALS. DON'T EAT FOOD OUT OF THE PACKAGE IT CAME WITH. RATHER MAKE PORTIONS OF IT AND WAIT TO ENJOY YOUR BEAUTIFUL DISH AFTER YOU ARE DONE WITH STYLING.

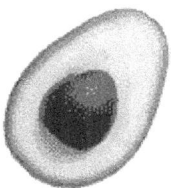

15

IF YOU ARE EASILY TEMPTED BY "UNHEALTHY" FOODS, YOU CAN PREPARE "FOOD PACKS" CONTAINING NUTRITIOUS STUFF LIKE NUTS, SLICED FRUITS AND VEGETABLES ETC. YOU CAN USE THE EMERGENCY PACKS WHENEVER YOU FIND YOURSELF HUNGRY.

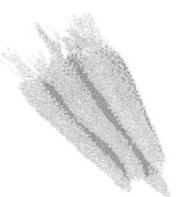

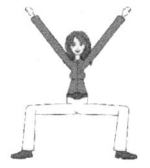

[WEIGHT LOSS TIPS 16 – 20]

16

TRY TO DO SOME WALKING OR OTHER EXERCISE BEFORE YOUR MAIN MEAL(S). AFTER EXERCISING YOU ARE LESS LIKELY TO MAKE A BAD FOOD CHOICE. YOU WILL ALSO EAT LESS.

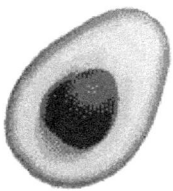

17

IT IS SAID THAT RED PEPPERS REDUCE A PERSON'S APPETITE AND HIS/HER NEED FOR FOOD. YOU CAN EAT THE PEPPERS IN THE MORNING AND THEY WILL REDUCE THE AMOUNT OF FOOD YOU WILL EAT THE REST OF THE DAY.

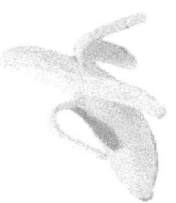

18

LOOKING FOR THE POWER OF FISH (ESPECIALLY SALMON OR TUNA) BUT

DON'T KNOW HOW TO COOK IT? TRY BUYING SOME PRE-COOKED FISH, WARM IT AND TRY IT.

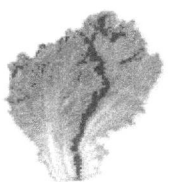

19

IT IS LIKELY THAT YOU EAT FASTER THAN YOU SHOULD. IF YOU EAT SLOWER YOU WILL EAT LESS FOOD. IT WILL ALSO MAKE YOU FEEL "FULL" EARLIER. TRY OPENING A CONVERSATION SO YOU EAT SLOWER.

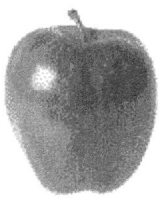

20

WHENEVER YOU NEED A BOOST IN YOUR METABOLISM, TRY DRINKING SOME TEA (FRESH TEA IF POSSIBLE) OR EAT SOME RED PEPPERS.

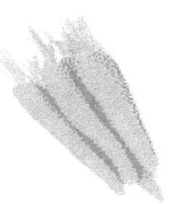

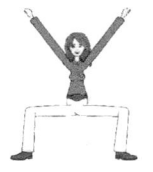

21

TAKE A GOOD SLEEP WHENEVER YOU FIND THE CHANCE (EVEN FOR 20' OR 30'). LACK OF SLEEP WILL CAUSE INCREASE IN THE LEVELS OF HORMONES IN THE BODY AND YOU'LL WANT TO EAT MORE.

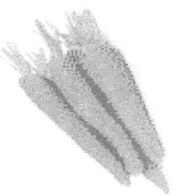

22

MOVE YOUR BODY WITH EVERY CHANCE. IT DOESN'T MATTER IF IT'S A SLOW MOVEMENT, A BIG OR A SMALL WALK. KEEP AN ATTITUDE OF A PERSON WHO WANTS TO BE IN THE "MOVE" ALL THE TIME.

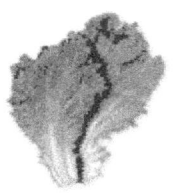

23

COFFEE IS A GREAT WAY TO GET ANTIOXIDANTS INTO YOUR BODY. YOU CAN TRY DECAF COFFEE WHICH IS A GREAT LOW-CALORIE DRINK AND GREAT FOR DIET.

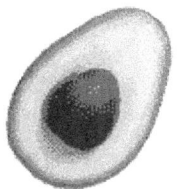

24

I KNOW DIPS ARE WONDERFUL AND SO ARE SAUCES. BUT IT WOULD BE WISER TO REPLACE FATTY DIPS LIKE A CREAM –BASED DIP WITH A NATURAL VEGETABLE DIP LIKE A BEAN-BASED DIP.

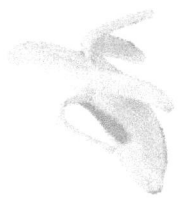

25

DOCTORS RECOMMED AT LEAST 10.000 STEPS EVERY DAY. YOU CAN BUY A PEDOMETER TO KEEP TRACK OF YOUR STEPS. YOU CAN FIND A PEDOMETER ON EBAY FOR A FEW DOLLARS.

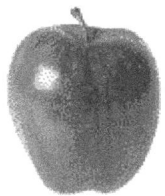

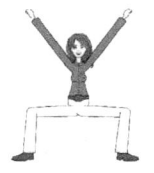

[WEIGHT LOSS TIPS
26 – 30]

26

IF YOU WANT TO INCREASE THE PLEASURE YOU RECEIVE FROM HEALTHY FOODS LIKE FRUITS, YOU CAN TRY A DIP SAUCE LIKE NATURAL APPLE-SAUCE.

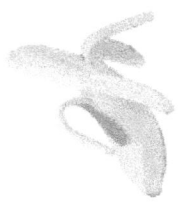

27

IF YOU PERFORM A STRENGTH STRAINING EXERCISE FOR 20', THREE OR FOUR TIMES PER WEEK, THEN YOU WILL BURN FOUR TIMES AS MANY CALORIES AS IF NO EXERCISE IS PERFORMED.

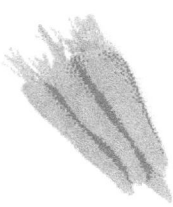

28

HAVE A GOAL OF LOSING WEIGHT (E.G. I WANT TO LOSE X POUNDS). KEEP REMINDING YOURSELF OF THIS GOAL WHENEVER YOU FIND YOURSELF TEMPTED BY UNHEALTHY FOODS.

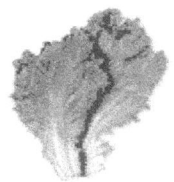

29

IF YOU WANT TO FEEL "FULL" WITH LESS FOOD, TRY EATING A SOUP OR DRINKING A NUTRITIOUS FRUIT JUICE. A SOUP WILL ALSO MAKE YOUR STOMACH STRONGER AND WELL LUBRICATED.

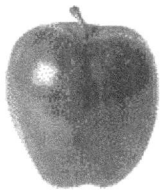

30

KEEP A JOURNAL OF YOUR WEIGHT-LOSS PROGRESS. WEIGH YOURSELF REGULARLY SO AS TO TRACK YOUR GOALS. FEEL HAPPY FOR EACH POUND YOU LOSE. KEEP IT GOING.

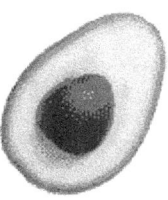

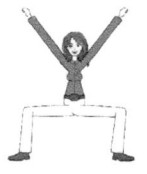

[WEIGHT LOSS TIPS 31 – 35]

31

USE SOME CINNAMON POWDER ON FRUITS LIKE BANANAS, APPLES, MELONS OR ORANGES. THIS WILL GIVE THE FRUIT A RICH *"DESSERT FEEL"* WITHOUT USING SUGAR AT ALL.

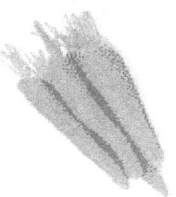

32

YOU MIGHT HAVE HEARD THIS. USE A GUM AND CHEW IT FOR AS MUCH TIME AS POSSIBLE. IT MIGHT MAKE YOU FEEL "FULL". OF COURSE THE GUM MUST BE SUGAR-FREE. THERE ARE ALL SORTS OF BEAUTIFULY FLAVORED, SUGAR-FREE GUMS.

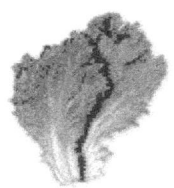

33

IT IS NOT WISE TO EAT IN FRONT OF A TV OR ON THE THEATER BECAUSE

YOU ARE BOUND TO CONSUME MORE FOOD AND THUS MORE CALORIES.

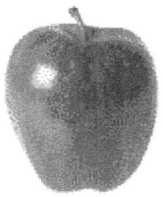

34

IF YOU FIND IT HARD TO START A DIET THEN MAKE A SMALL FIRST STEP. FOR EXAMPLE GO BUY SOME FRUITS OR SOME NEW WALKING SHOES. YOU GOT MORE CHANCES TO FOLLOW THROUGH IF YOU MAKE A SMALL STEP...

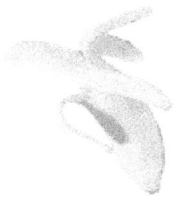

35

AVOID EATING FAT-FREE FOODS BECAUSE THESE ARE OVER-PROCESSED AND THEY CONTAIN LARGE PORTIONS OF SALT, SUGAR AND SODIUM INSTEAD OF THE ORIGINAL FATS.

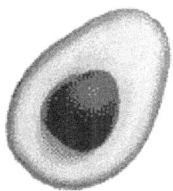

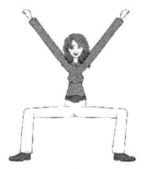

36

REPLACE FULL FAT MILK AT BREAKFAST WITH A NATURAL JUICE LIKE ORANGE JUICE. IT WILL BOOST YOUR ENERGY LEVELS AND IT WILL ALSO PROTECT YOUR BODY. SKIM MILK IS NOT A BAD CHOICE THOUGH.

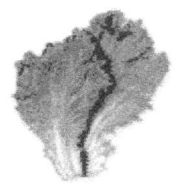

37

EXTRA LOW CALORIE DRINKS ARE NOT AS GOOD AS IT IS PRESENTED. I AM NOT SAYING YOU SHOULD AVOID THEM, JUST DON'T OVER-USE THEM.

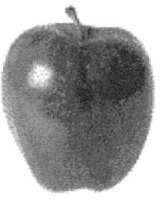

38

IF YOU ARE DESPERATE FOR A SNACK THEN TRY EATING FRUITS LIKE PEARS, PEACHES OR BERRIES AND THEY WILL HELP YOU LOWER YOUR APPETITE.

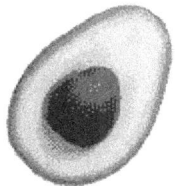

39

IF YOU ARE SERIOUS ABOUT WEIGHT LOSS THEN REPLACE ALL SUGAR BEVERAGES (AND WHY NOT SUGAR-FREE AS WELL) WITH **PURE WATER**. THIS IS THE BEST GIFT YOU CAN GIVE TO YOURSELF. IT WILL HELP YOU LOSE WEIGHT EASIER AND FASTER.

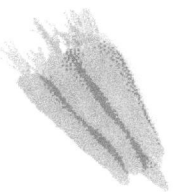

40

VEGETABLES SHOULD BE AN IMPORTANT PART OF YOUR DIET (IF YOU WANT TO LOSE WEIGHT EASILY). ALWAYS HAVE VEGETABLES IN YOUR KITCHEN. YOU CAN ALSO FREEZE THEM.

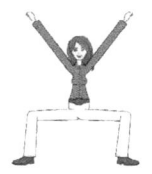

41

SPEAKING OF FROZEN VEGETABLES, YOU CAN LOOK IN THE FROZEN FOOD DEPARTMENT FOR FROZEN SOY BEANS. IT IS CONSIDERED A GREAT SNACK AND LOW COST.

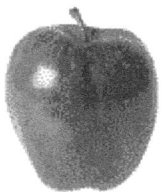

42

MANY PEOPLE GET TOO RELAXED DURING WEEKENDS BUT LOSING WEIGHT SHOULD BE A 7-DAYS PER WEEK CHALLENGE. FIND SOME EXCEPTIONAL ACTIVITY OR EXERCISE FOR WEEKENDS.

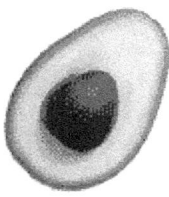

43

SAVE TIME AND MONEY BY BUYING FOOD IN BULK AND THEN FREEZE THE ITEMS. YOU SHOULD GENERALLY AVOID RED MEATS AND REPLACE

THEM WITH LEAN PROTEIN LIKE FRESH OR FROZEN CHICKEN BREASTS. FISH IS ANOTHER GREAT ALTERNATIVE.

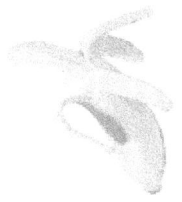

44

EAT FRUITS AND VEGETABLES THAT ARE IN SEASON. THIS WAY YOU WILL ENJOY THEM MORE. YOU WILL ALSO EXPECT THEIR COMING WHEN IT IS THE RIGHT SEASON. THERE ARE PLENTY OF VEGETABLES AND FRUITS FOR ALL SEASONS.

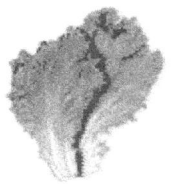

45

IS FOOD YOUR ONLY PLEASURE? WHY NOT TRY TO ACCOMPANY IT WITH SOME OTHER, ACTIVITY (E.G. SPORTS, GYM) THAT WILL ALSO HELP YOU BURN CALORIES? DANCING (MUSIC) IS A ANOTHER GREAT OPTION...

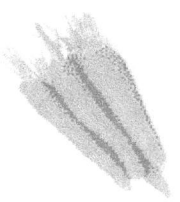

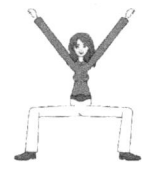

[WEIGHT LOSS TIPS 46 – 50]

46

SCIENTISTS SAY THAT PROTEIN IS MORE SATISFYING AND FULFILLING THAN FATS OR CARBS. SO, IT WOULD BE WISE TO ALWAYS HAVE SOME LEAN PROTEIN HANDY. EAT SMALL PORTIONS WITH EVERY MEAL.

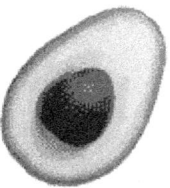

47

(AGAIN) YOU CAN EAT SOUPS WITH EVERY CHANCE. THEY WILL MAKE YOU FEEL FULL EASIER AND THEY WILL GIVE YOU A LOT OF NUTRIENTS. A NICE VEGETABLE SOUP IS NOT A DIFFICULT FOOD TO PREPARE.

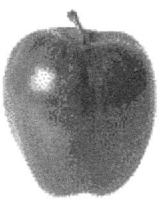

48

AVOID JUNK FOOD (FAST FOOD). IF YOU CAN'T RESIST THE TEMPTATION THEN TRY TO FIGHT IT BY GOING AND BUYING SOME FRUITS AND VEGETABLES.

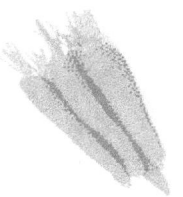

49

IF YOU USE THE TABLE WHERE YOU EAT IN YOUR KITCHEN FOR OTHER ACTIVITIES, YOU MIGHT BE TEMPTED TO EAT SOMETHING WHILE PERFORMING THESE ACTIVITIES. USE THIS TABLE ONLY FOR EATING.

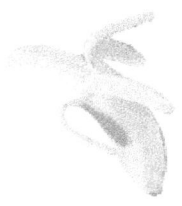

50

BREAKFAST IS THE MOST IMPORTANT MEAL OF THE DAY. SO, HAVE A GOOD BREAKFAST EVERY DAY AND STAY STRONG THE REST OF THE DAY. YOU WILL LIKELY EAT LESS OF THE OTHER MEALS OF THE DAY.

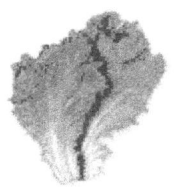

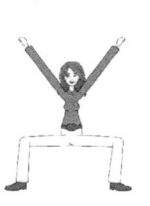

[WEIGHT LOSS TIPS 51– 55]

51

WHEN MEASURING YOUR WEIGHT, USE A TAPE MEASURE INSTEAD OF A SCALE. YOUR GOAL SHOULD BE 33" INCHES FOR WOMEN AND 35" INCHES FOR MEN. THAT IS 84 CENTIMETRES FOR WOMEN AND 89 CENTIMETRES FOR MEN.

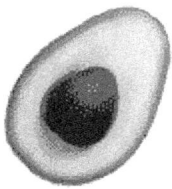

52

(AGAIN) FISH OIL AND ESPECIALLY SALMON AND TUNA OILS ARE GREAT FAT BURNERS. SO, CONSUME FISH WITH EVERY CHANCE. COMBINE IT WITH SOME EXERCISE (E.G. SOME WALKING) AND YOU WILL START LOSING WEIGHT IMMEDIATELY.

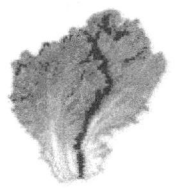

53

YOU CAN TRY EATING A NICE FRUIT BEFORE EVERY MEAL (ESPECIALLY

THE MAIN MEAL) AND IT WILL REDUCE THE AMOUNT OF FOOD YOU CONSUME DURING THE MEAL AND LATER FOR THE REST OF THE DAY.

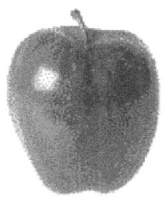

54

IF YOU ARE LIKE ME YOU LIKE PASTA. IN FACT, YOU LOVE IT. BUT YOU CAN REPLACE REGULAR PASTA WITH WHOLE WHEAT PASTA AND IT WILL MAKE YOU FEEL MORE "FULL".

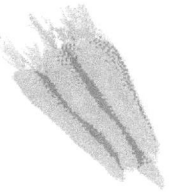

55

HERE ARE 5 FOODS THAT CAN SECRETLY HELP YOU LOSE WEIGHT ESPECIALLY IF YOU FOLLOW A GENERALLY HEALTHY LIFE-STYLE: HONEY, SKIM MILK, BANANAS, BERRIES, AND PSYLLIUM SEED HUSKS.

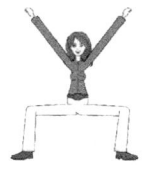

[WEIGHT LOSS TIPS 56 – 60]

56

A RECENT RESEARCH SHOWED THAT IF YOU EAT EGGS IN THE MORNING, YOU ARE LIKELY TO EAT LESS FOOD THAN IF YOU HAD A CARB-BASED BREAKFAST.

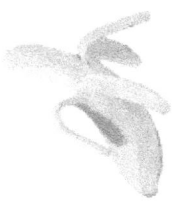

57

WHEN SHOPPING FOR GROCERY ALWAYS PAY ATTENTION TO THE INGREDIENT LABELS FOR EVERYTHING YOU BUY. AVOID HIGHLY PROCESSED FOOD AND FOOD WITH HIGH PERCENTAGE OF FATS/SUGAR/SALT.

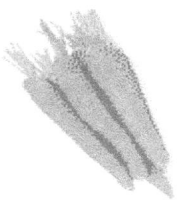

58

TRY THE MEDITERRANEAN DIET. IT IS WELL KNOW FOR ITS HEART STRENGTHENING QUALITIES AND FOR BETTER WEIGHT LOSS RESULTS. IT

IS ALSO SIMPLE TO FOLLOW. START FROM EXTRA VIRGIN OLIVE OIL AND THE PREPARATION OF A GREEK SALAD.

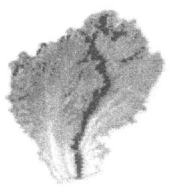

59

YOU KNOW WHAT TO AVOID, RIGHT? ALL THESE FOODS THAT TASTE SO GOOD OF COURSE!. YOU HAVE TO EAT AS LITTLE AS YOU CAN OF THEM. FOODS LIKE CREAM CHEESE AND BUTTER. INSTEAD TRY TO FIND HEALTHY ALTERNATIVES. TRY PEANUT OR ALMOND BUTTER FOR EXAMPLE.

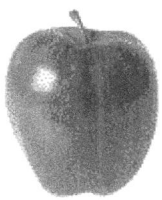

60

WHEN YOU ARE READY TO ORDER IN A RESTAURANT, ASK THE WAITER WHAT ARE THE HEALTHIEST OPTIONS IN THE MENU.

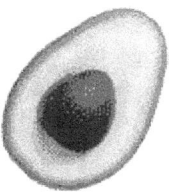

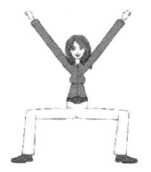

61

INSTEAD OF CALCULATING POUNDS/KILOGRAMS AIM FOR A CERTAIN DRESS SIZE OR WAIST MEASUREMENT (REMEMBER THE MEASUREMENT TAPE?). DON'T BE OBSESSED WITH SCALE NUMBERS AND POUNDS/KILOS AS THEY MIGHT MAKE YOU MORE NERVOUS.

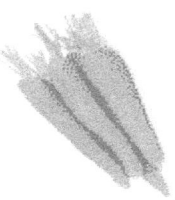

62

YOU CAN CARRY YOUR PERSONAL *"SNACK-BOX"* AT WORK SO YOU WILL NOT BE TEMPTED BY A QUICK UNHEALTHY SNACK OR A CANDY FROM YOUR COLLEAGUE'S DESK. PUT DRIED FRUITS, NUTS IN FIXED PORTIONS INSIDE THE BOX.

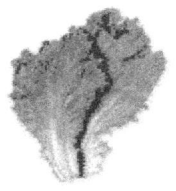

63

IF YOU WANT TO GIVE AN EXTRA TASTE-BOOST TO YOUR MORNING

EGGS OR EVENING CHICKEN, THEN ADD SOME RED CHILLI PEPPER SAUCE.

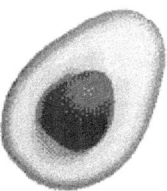

64

IT IS BETTER TO COOK YOUR OWN FOOD OR FIND A SOURCE FOR HEALTHY FOOD THAN EATING PRE-MADE MEALS WHICH NEED THE USE OF A MICROWAVE FOR EXAMPLE. IF YOU MUST USE MICROWAVE, CHOOSE CHICKEN FILLETS, VEGETABLE BURGERS OR OTHER VEGETABLES YOU PREFER.

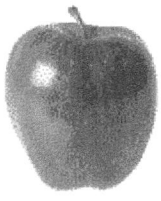

65

USE YOUR FAVORITES SPICES TO BOOST THE FLAVOR OF YOUR LEFT-OVERS FROM YESTERDAY'S DINNER. E.G. SOME MUSTARD, CHILLI PEPPER POWDER, CURRY POWDER ETC.

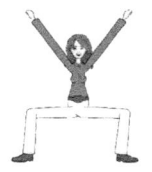

66

COLORS PLAY AN IMPORTANT PART IN A PERSON'S DIET. A VARIETY OF BRIGHT COLORS MUST BE USED (CONSUMED IN FOODS). FOR EXAMPLE YOU CAN PREPARE A RAINBOW SALAD WITH ALL SORTS OF COLORS AND INGREDIENTS.

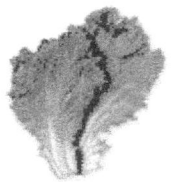

67

DO YOU WANT AN ALTERNATIVE FOR MEAT? I GOT 2 FOR YOU. THE FIRST IS BEANS. THE SECOND IS MUSHROOMS. THEY CAN PLAY THE ROLE OF A BEEF FILLET EASILY.

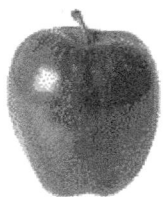

68

A NICE YOGHURT LOADED WITH PROTEIN WILL MAKE AN UNBEATABLE SNACK. AGAIN, CHOOSE ORIGINAL, UNSWEETENED YOGHURT. IT WILL

PROVIDE YOU WITH NATURAL PROBIOTICS AND CALSIUM WHICH IS GREAT FOR THE SKELETAL SYSTEM.

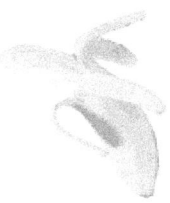

69

BEFORE EXERCISING (OF ANY KIND), TRY A NICE GREEK YOGHURT FOR MORE STRENGTH AND BODY ENERGY. TRY THE ONES WITH SHEEP'S AND GOAT'S MILK (REMEMBER READING THE INGREDIENTS IN THE LABEL?)

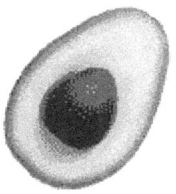

70

FIX YOUR WARDROBE SO IT MATCHES YOUR GOALS. AS YOU LOSE WEIGHT, YOU MIGHT WANT TO DONATE YOUR OLD CLOTHES THAT DON'T FIT AND MAKE A COMMITMENT NOT TO GO BACK TO BEING OVER-WEIGHT AGAIN!

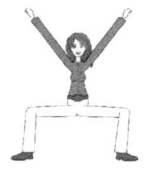

[WEIGHT LOSS TIPS
71 – 75]

71

USE MEDITATION AND VISUALIZATION TO IMAGINE EXCESSIVE WEIGHT BEING THROWN AWAY FROM YOU AND BEING RECYCLED SOMEWHERE IN OUTER SPACE WHERE IT CAN'T HURT ANYONE OR ANYTHING...

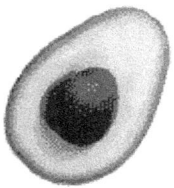

72

EXPERIMENT WITH A PASTA-LESS SPAGHETTI. REPLACE IT WITH SLICED ZUCCHINI OR OTHER VEGETABLES OF YOUR CHOICE ALONG WITH THE SPAGHETTI SAUCE. YOU CAN ALSO ADD FRESH MUSHROOMS AND OREGANO.

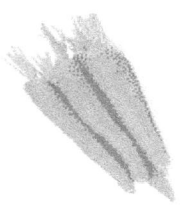

73

BY MEASURING THE PORTIONS OF MEAT YOU COOK AND/OR EAT YOU

CREATE A NICE HABIT OF EATING FIXED PORTIONS. MOST OF THE TIMES IT'S NOT WHAT YOU EAT, BUT HOW MUCH YOU EAT.-

74

IF YOU ARE USED TO FAST FOOD (CONSIDERED JUNK FOOD) THEN YOU CONSUME A LOT OF SALT. YOU CAN BALANCE THIS BY DRINKING WATER. ALSO, REMEMBER THAT IF YOU FOLLOW A MORE HEALTHY DIET (LESS JUNK), YOU WILL BE ABLE TO EASILY RECOGNIZE THE NATURAL SALTS IN FOODS.

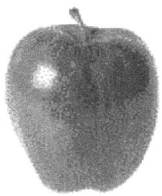

75

DID YOU KNOW YOU CAN SAVE UP TO 100 CALORIES IF YOU REPLACE MAYONNAISE WITH PLAIN MUSTARD IN A HOME-MADE SANDWICH?

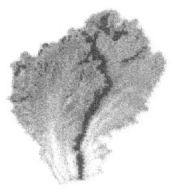

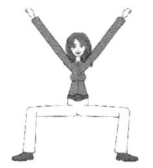

76

IF YOU CAN, MAKE IT A HABIT NOT TO EAT AFTER 8 O'CLOCK IN THE EVENING. IF YOU CANNOT RESIST THE TEMPTATION AND YOU FEEL HUNGRY, EAT A FRUIT OR SOME YOGHURT. SAVE YOUR APPETITE FOR THE NEXT MORNING (BREAKFAST).

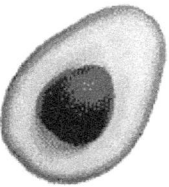

77

IF YOU FIND YOURSELF IN THE "FLOW" OF LOSING WEIGHT THEN PERFORM AN EXERCISE OR INCREASE THE DURATION OF YOUR REGULAR EXERCISE BY 5' MINUTES.

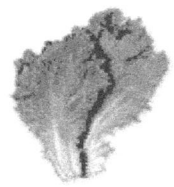

78

HERBS CAN REALLY BOOST THE QUALITY AND TASTE OF A MEAL/FOOD. FIND THE ONES YOU ENJOY THE MOST AND USE THEM FRESH (OR

DRIED) IN YOUR RECIPES. MAYBE YOU SHOULD PRODUCE YOUR OWN HERBS IN A SMALL SELF-MADE HERBAL GARDEN!

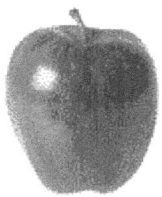

79

I HAVE NOTICED MANY RECIPES WHERE ORIGINAL CREAM IS REPLACED WITH SILKEN TOFU. I SUGGEST YOU TRY IT TO YOUR OWN WEIGHT LOSS RECIPES.

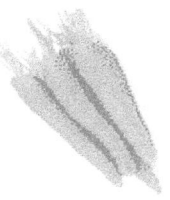

80

(AGAIN) START USING/EATING EXTRA VIRGIN OLIVE OIL. YOU CAN CONSUME IT IN A VARIETY OF WAYS. TO TRY THE QUALITY OF THE OIL, POUR A DROP IN YOUR FINGER AND THEN TASTE IT (WITH THE EDGE OF YOUR TONGUE).

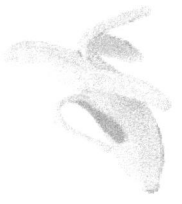

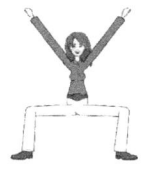

81

IF YOU ARE LUCKY ENOUGH TO HAVE A SIGNIFIVANT OTHER AND IT HAPPENS SO YOU ARE BOTH ON A DIET, THEN TRY TO PACK/PREPARE EACH OTHER SNACKS (REMEMBER *"SNACK BOXES"*?). THIS IS ALSO A GREAT WAY TO SURPRISE EACH OTHER.

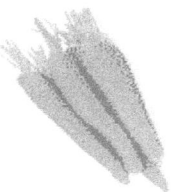

82

A WELL GUARDED WEIGHT LOSS SECRET IS… AVOCADOS! YES THIS FRUIT IS POWERFUL, HIGH IN HEALTHY FATS AND FIBERS. *"A WISH COME TRUE"* FOR PEOPLE ON A DIET.-

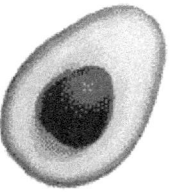

83

OTHER FOODS THAT CAN GIVE YOU A FEELING OF A "FULL" STOMACH

ARE: ASPARAGUS, OLIVES, LOW SODIUM SOY AND... MUSHROOMS (AGAIN)!

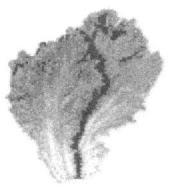

84

FIND AND KEEP A GOOD POSTURE AT WORK AND WHEN YOU SIT ON A CHAIR ETC. THIS WAY YOU WILL BURN EXTRA CALORIES TRYING TO MAINTAIN THE POSITION. SMART?

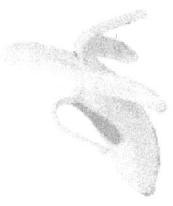

85

AN ALTERNATIVE FOR POTATO CHIPS (FRENCH FRIES OR FRIED POTATOES ONE OF THE MOST POPULAR FOODS WORLDWIDE) IS "BAKED APPLE SLICES" ☺

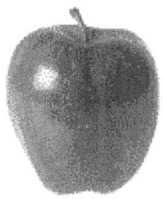

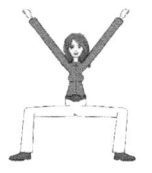

86

DRINK A LOT OF WATER (AT LEAST 10 GLASSES PER DAY) AND FOODS CONTAINING WATER LIKE TOMATOES, MELONS, CUCUMBERS ETC. ALSO JUICY FRUITS LIKE ORANGES, CHERRIES ETC.

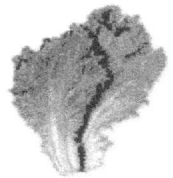

87

AVOID TASTY BUT UNHEALTHY APPETIZERS IN RESTAURANTS. MOST OF THEM ARE FRIED ANYWAY... REPLACE YOUR STARTERS WITH A NICE VEGETABLE SALAD.

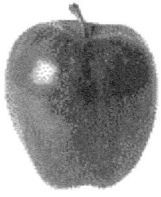

88

WOULD YOU LIKE A FOOD THAT IS RICH IN MAGNESIUM AND IT WILL ALSO LOWER YOUR BLOOD PRESSURE? HERE IT IS: **PUMPKIN SEEDS** OR **SUNFLOWER SEEDS** (BOTH UNSALTED).

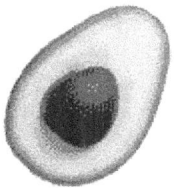

89

USE THE STAIRS, THE PERFECT WORKOUT AS ADM TTED BY MAIN TRAINERS. YOU CAN FIND STAIRS EVERYWHERE. SO, NEXT TIME YOU SEE THEM, DON'T TAKE THE ELEVATOR.

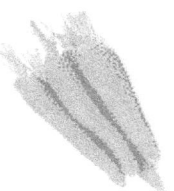

90

WHEN YOU ARE TIRED IT IS MORE LIKELY TO BE HUNGRY AS WELL. SO INSTEAD OF EATING SOME BAD FOOD, TAKE A QUICK S_EEP (EVEN 20' OR 30' MINUTES).

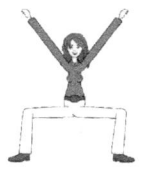

[WEIGHT LOSS TIPS
91 – 95]

91

A GOOD WEIGHT LOSS ADVICE, IS TO SHARE YOUR GOALS WITH YOUR FRIENDS AND FAMILY. LET THEM KNOW YOUR COMMITMENT TO LOSING A CERTAIN AMOUNT OF POUNDS/KILOS IN A CERTAIN AMOUNT OF TIME.

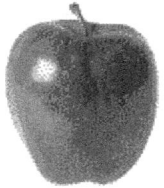

92

"RESISTANCE BANDS" ARE A GREAT WORKOUT (FOR BOTH MEN AND WOMEN) IF YOU WANT TO LOSE EXTRA POUNDS. JUST USE THIS TOOL WITH CONSISTENCY AND CARE.

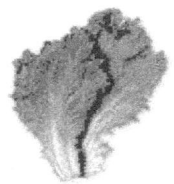

93

SALAD DRESSINGS ARE PACKED WITH CALORIES. INSTEAD USE SOME

LEMON JUICE AND/OR VINEGAR, EXTRA VIRGIN OLIVE OIL AND SOME HERBS LIKE OREGANO ETC.

94

TRY THIS: TAKE A 30'' SECOND BREAK WHILE YOU EAT A MEAL. MAKE AN EVALUATION OF JUST HOW HUNGRY YOU ARE BEFORE YOU RETURN TO YOUR DISH...

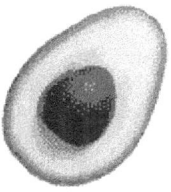

95

GET TO KNOW *"QUINOA"* – A POWERFUL FOOD – PACKED WITH LOTS OF GOODIES FOR YOUR OVERALL BODY SYSTEM. QUINOA IS A GRAIN FULL OF QUALITIES. DISCOVER IT.

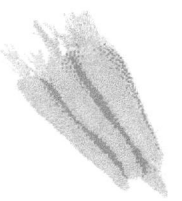

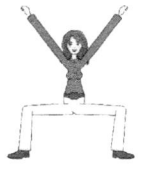

96

TAKE MAYONNAISE AND CHEESE OFF AND EAT A SANDWITCH WITH 250 CALORIES LESS WHEN YOU ARE IN A RESTAURANT.

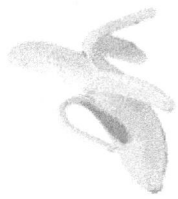

97

IF YOU WANT TO KEEP TRACK OF YOUR PROGRESS (REMEMBER YOUR JOURNAL?), THEN TAKE A PHOTO OF YOU IN FRONT OF THE MIRROR EACH DAY.

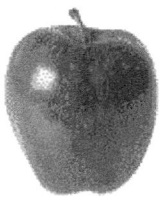

98

IF YOU WANT TO AVOID EATING A SECOND PLATE FROM YOUR MEAL YOU SHOULD PACK WHAT WAS LEFT FROM THE MEAL BEFORE YOU SIT ON THE TABLE TO EAT. THIS WAY YOU WILL NOT TEMPTED TO EAT MORE.

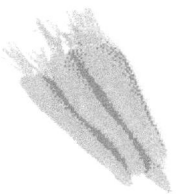

99

ONE GOOD EXERCISE IF YOU ARE A STARTER IN WEIGHT LOSS MEDITATION IS YOGA. IT IS AN IDEAL WORKOUT IF YOU ARE ON A DIET AND NOT THAT HARD TO LEARN AND APPLY.

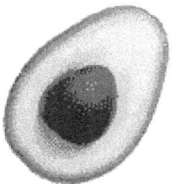

100

USE YOUR FREEZER TO FREEZE VEGETABLES AND FRUITS SO YOU CAN EAT THEM (AS SPECIAL DELIGHTS) WHEN THEY GO OUT OF SEASON. YOU CAN FREEZE GRAPES, BERRIES OR PEPPERS AND TOMATOES.

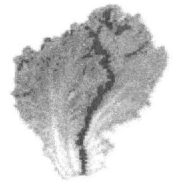

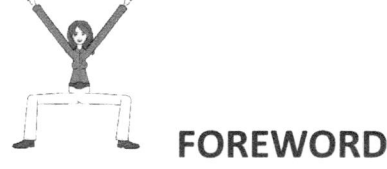

FOREWORD

SO THAT WAS ALL!

I HOPE YOU ENJOYED MY **WEIGHT LOSS TIPS** BUT MOST OF ALL I HOPE YOU WILL PUT THEM TO ACTION AND START LOSING WEIGHT AS SOON AS POSSIBLE.

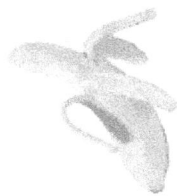

AS YOU MIGHT HAVE UNDERSTOOD, LOSING WEIGHT IS NOT JUST A PHYSICAL PROCESS. IT IS ALSO A SPIRITUAL PROCESS AND THIS MEANS THAT YOU CAN LOSE WEIGHT USING SPIRITUAL EXERCISES LIKE YOGA MEDITATION (MENTIONED IN THE WEIGHT LOSS TIPS).

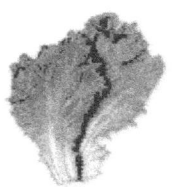

I SUPPOSE YOU WANTED MORE TIPS OR MORE CONTENT TO READ BUT HERE'S HOW YOU SHOULD USE THIS BOOK. USE EVERY TIP AS *"FOOD FOR THOUGHT"* AND EXPAND EACH OF THE HUNDRED CONCEPTS IN YOUR MIND.

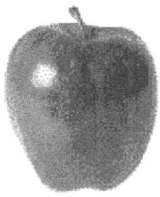

ALSO, TO EXPLORE MORE, LOOK AT THE PROMOTIONS IN THE FOLLOWING PAGES.

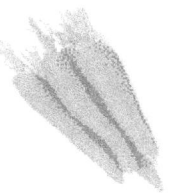

IF YOU LIKED THIS BOOK THEN PLEASE TAKE THE TIME TO LEAVE A POSITIVE REVIEW ON AMAZON. THIS WILL BE THE GREATER GIFT FOR THE AUTHOR AND THE BEST WAY TO BLOW US TO HEAVENS!

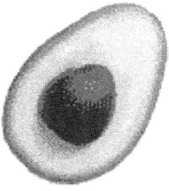

I WISH YOU ALL SUCCESS IN YOUR WEIGHT LOSS GOALS.- SO BE IT.-

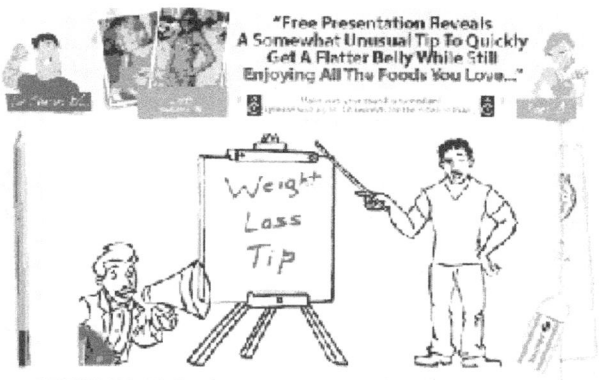

"...FREE PRESENTATION REVEALS A SOMEWHAT UNUSUAL TIP TO QUICKLY GET A FLATTER BELLY WHILE STILL ENJOYING ALL THE FOODS YOU LOVE..." **VISIT THIS LINK:**

http://hyperdeals.biz/go/10/

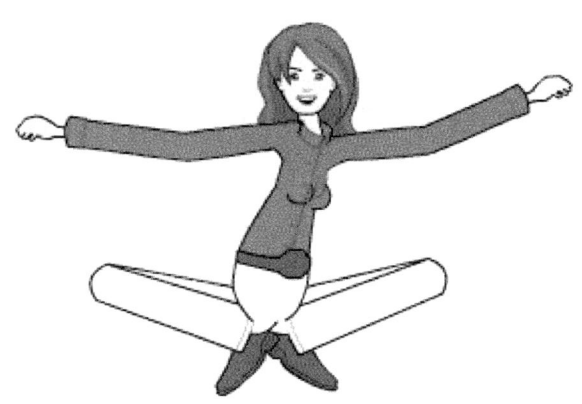

CREDITS

FIRST AND FOREMOST I WANT TO THANK MY PUBLISHER LAZAROS GEORGOULAS WHO MADE THIS LITTLE BOOK A REALITY FOR ME. THANK YOU FROM THE BOTTOM OF MY HEART FOR MAKING MY LIFE EASIER AND HAPPIER!

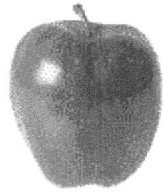

NEXT I WANT TO THANK DR. OZMAN BARSELL PHD WHO ADDED HIS WISDOM IN MY TIPS

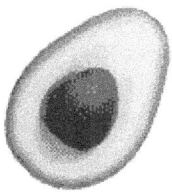

ILLUSTRATIONS CREATED BY MARIA MARKELLA AND LAZAROS GEORGOULAS

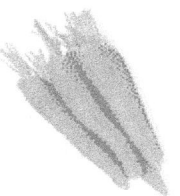

THE AUTHOR CANNOT GUARANTEE THAT THE TIPS WILL MAKE YOU LOSE WEIGHT ALTHOUGH SHE PUT ALL HER EFFORTS TO PRESENT VALID ADVICE AND INFORMATION. LOSING WEIGHT IS A PERSONAL CHALLENGE AND SUCCESS CAN ONLY BE GUARANTEED BY YOU.

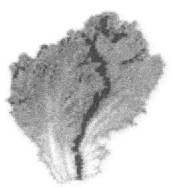

YOU ARE FREE TO LEND THIS BOOK TO WHOEVER NEEDS TO LOSE WEIGHT. YOU ARE FREE TO SHARE IT OR EVEN ADAPT IT.

THE IMAGES OF THE 5 FOODS IN THIS BOOK WERE NOT SELECTED BY LUCK. :)

THE END???

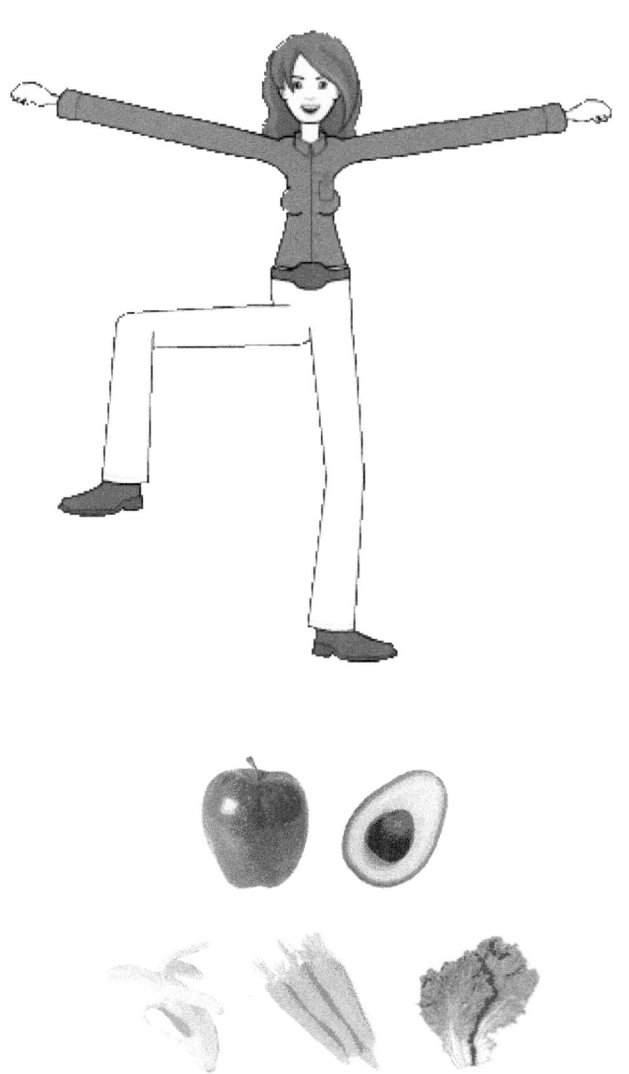